Pregnancy: The Ultimate Pregnancy Handbook for First Time Moms

Contents

Introduction

I want to thank you and congratulate you for downloading the book, *"Pregnancy: The Ultimate Pregnancy Handbook for First Time Moms"*.

This book contains proven steps and strategies on how to prepare for pregnancy especially if you're first time mom.

Pregnancy is serious business. Yes, having a baby is a blessing, but as mentioned earlier, it can also be pretty tiring -- and scary! Nevertheless, many moms would agree on this – nothing beats the joy of conceiving, carrying a baby in the womb for nine months, and giving birth. You can bask in that joy if you are well-prepared, which is why I wrote this book.

The book also contains important things you need to know and expect during all three trimesters of your pregnancy, the kind of diet you need to follow, and how you can keep yourself safe and healthy during the entire term of your pregnancy.

You do not have to go into pregnancy blindly when proven tips and helpful pieces of advice are within your reach.

Thanks again for downloading this book. I hope you enjoy it!

The information herein is offered for informational purposes solely, and is universal as so. The presentation of the information is without contract or any type of guarantee assurance.

The trademarks that are used are without any consent, and the publication of the trademark is without permission or backing by the trademark owner. All trademarks and brands within this book are for clarifying purposes only and are the owned by the owners themselves, not affiliated with this document.

Chapter 1: A Guide To First-Time Moms

So you want to be a good mom? Don't worry. You will be! You just need to know what to expect. This chapter is all about letting you know what you're in for – and while it's natural to be nervous about the whole thing, preparing for it will ensure that you and your baby will be healthy and happy.

First-time moms are in for a different kind of experience once a baby enters their life. It doesn't even start after delivery – it starts once you see those two pink lines confirming that you have a *life* in your womb. You'll experience a slew of emotions -- a mixture of excitement, happiness, fear, and many others. It's normal to be nervous. You'd even find yourself worrying a bit about pains during delivery. Aside from that, the imagination of a first-time mom usually goes into overdrive. You might find yourself thinking about the foreseeable future and worrying about whether you can give your baby a good life.

Emotions run high and you'll tend to be extra sensitive during pregnancy, thanks to hormones, which is why you really need to understand your needs and how your body works, and the changes that will occur – from the subtle to the not-so-subtle. If you do that, first-time pregnancy and parenting will be manageable.

The joys of pregnancy and parenthood are overwhelming, but pregnancies also come with a need for a great deal of work, patience, love, support, and understanding. Here are some of the challenges, reminders, and pieces of advice that you should consider so you will enjoy this new stage of your life.

What To Expect When You're Expecting

Conception, pregnancy, childbirth, and child rearing are no walk in the park. It's easy to say you want to have a baby, but once the baby is there, you discover how hard reality bites. Here are some expectations you need to be ready for:

The Pains of Childcare

Childcare will definitely burn your energy especially the first few years, and more so, the first few months. You should be ready for sleep interruptions during the night. You will get exhausted during the day may not have enough energy to look after the baby at night. Once you're back to work, you have that to worry about too. You might want to consider asking for a more flexible shift at work. If that isn't possible, hire a nanny who can look after your child. It is going to be worth it. Nothing compares to the feeling of waking up and staying late just staring at the little angel.

Set Your Priorities

Once you're confirmed that a baby is on the way, it's time to readjust your priorities. This is the first thing you have to remember – you should not try to be a superwoman. You don't have to make sure that your house is spotless, that you serve well-planned healthy meals all the time, maintain your relationships with all friends and work full-time all while taking care of your baby. You have to be realistic about what can be done without stretching yourself too thin. Find out what's more important to you and build your schedule around that. Perhaps, you don't have to keep the place spotless. Perhaps, eating out a few nights a week is okay. You don't even have to completely stick to a rigid schedule. Part of being a parent is thinking on your feet.

Establish a support system

You are going to be your child's anchor but it doesn't hurt to get support from other people, as well. Remember what they say about how it takes a village to raise a child. You don't need a literal village to help you out – you can just ask friends or family not exactly for help but for support. Ask someone over for dinner so you and your child can get some socialization with people other than each other. Also, contrary to popular belief, you can actually endear yourself to someone by asking for help – especially if it's something as easy as help with moving the couch. Even something as simple as calling your own parents to talk about how things are with your child is a good way to establish that support system.

Stay Healthy

Motherhood is going to take a lot of energy so staying fit is important. You should never forget to take care of yourself. That way, you can take care of your child and their needs. Motherhood is a 24/7 job, and you can't afford to get sick or fall to a serious condition because a tiny human being is now dependent on you. Still, you do need some time off to take care of your personal needs, which is why you'll need a readjustment of priorities and a decent support system.

It's challenging – but rewarding -- to be a first-time mom. There will be ups and downs, but if you are determined to take on the challenge, you'll find that it can be fun and exciting – even wondrous at times. Parenthood becomes even more meaningful once you start teaching your child the value of respect, love, and responsibility – and just how to be a good human being in general.

Chapter 2: Things You Need to Consider When Preparing for Pregnancy

When you get pregnant, your body goes through major changes. You might think that all the changes hormones brought during puberty were enough to make you crazy but just wait until they get to work during your pregnancy! Hence, it's crucial that prepare physically and also mentally. The physical aspect is a given, of course. After all, you'll be nourishing a life inside you. But you see, pregnancy is bound to catapult you into something you may not be quite prepared for. Yes, you expect to get pregnant someday and you might have even been fervently wishing for it. Whatever the case may be, expectation can be quite different from reality; thus, the need to prepare yourself mentally.

You may need to consider your career. This consideration goes hand-in-hand with finances, which is also a crucial part of being a parent. You'd want to make sure that your baby's needs are taken care of. There are some important questions that you will need to ask yourself. How quickly do you intend to get back to work? How do you manage your career and a baby? Pregnancy doesn't come free. In fact, it is expensive. Can you afford to leave your job and risk going through mental stress while trying to think of how you can make ends meet and sustain your pregnancy? Bear in mind the medical bills, the cost of having the baby, baby needs and supplies, and even your own needs. That's why it's important to prepare yourself mentally for the pregnancy challenge.

The next thing you need to work on is preparing your body for pregnancy. As mentioned in the beginning, your body will undergo changes before, during, and after the pregnancy. Therefore, it's important to make sure that your body stays healthy through the entire process. The first thing you need to do is to optimize your weight. You want to enter your pregnancy in the pink of health, so you need to ensure that you are neither overweight nor underweight. Start maintaining a healthy diet. Consult your obstetrician for help on this regard or ask her if she can refer you to a nutritionist. If you were a smoker, now's the best time to quit.

Smoking can lead to low birth weight for your baby, premature labor, and a plethora of other health problems for both you and the baby, not to mention that it can make conceiving a baby difficult in the first place because of the fertility problems it brings. Avoid cigarettes and secondhand smoke.

You may also prepare your body for the pregnancy by taking supplements and prenatal vitamins. Vitamins rich in folic acid and iron are vital, and you would do well to take these in large quantities once pregnant.

The next chapter will provide you with a close-up look on the different stages of pregnancy.

Chapter 3: The Three Stages of Pregnancy

Welcoming a baby to your life is one of the most exciting life experiences for a woman. Many await it with great eagerness and are overjoyed once they confirm the pregnancy.

Of course, having a clear understanding of the different stages of pregnancy can make a huge difference in how a mother-to-be faces the next nine months. There's really no need to panic even if this is your first time. There are many helpful tips and ideas that can make the upcoming months more comfortable.

To get a good overview of pregnancy, allow me to share a few key details about its three stages.

The First Trimester

The first trimester is composed of the next three months following the last menstrual cycle.

This is the stage where you will often experience morning sickness. Breast heaviness, tiredness, and frequent urination may even become daily occurrences at this point.

To reduce the tendencies of nausea, the recommended solution is to take small meals frequently. During this period, walking is a good exercise and watching your diet plays a vital role. Observe your weight and do not overeat to avoid possible problems in the future.

The baby, on the other hand, will be about 2.5 cm in length and 2g in weight. Eyes, nose, and ears will also start to form during this stage. Seeing him grow during every visit to the doctor is possibly one of the thrilling experiences of motherhood.

The Second Trimester

The second trimester is composed of the fourth to sixth months. Others call this period as the most enjoyable among the three stages of pregnancy.

Morning sickness ends during this is the time and you will feel more energetic. You will also be more open when it comes to talking about your pregnancy with others. On top of that, your appetite and sexual drive will significantly grow. Be warned, however, that the urge to urinate will increase significantly. It is also common to experience lower back pain and swelling feet. Kegel exercises are recommended in this trimester.

During these months, the baby will be about 10 inches and 300g. The heart will be completely developed by this time. Fingernails and toenails will start to appear plus the baby will begin getting small amount of hair, including eyelashes and eyebrows.

Third Trimester

The seventh to ninth months of pregnancy fall under the third trimester. Some refer to this as the "slowest" and most challenging of all the pregnancy stages. With a bigger tummy, frequent fatigue, and sleepless nights, you will probably be more restless at this point. Strictly obeying the doctor's counsels is crucial during this period. Certain exercises will probably be recommended to reduce the pains of your labor, especially if this is your first baby.

The baby will already be 16 inches and 2100g. All the body parts, organs and systems will be fully complete.

By understanding the developmental stages of pregnancy, you will know the appropriate diet and exercise to help your baby become healthy. Developing a pregnancy diet and following it religiously can be for your advantage.

Consult with your doctor often if you have specific medical conditions that need to be treated during pregnancy. Never take any medicine unless your physician personally recommended it. Supplements and vitamins may also be given for you to gain health benefits.

Chapter 4: Pregnancy Discomforts You Should be Aware Of

Being pregnant is no joke. You'll undergo a series of major changes in their bodies, most of which are going to be really uncomfortable – and some are even downright painful. Your feet swells, your back aches, you become emotionally unstable, your hormones fluctuate, and your appetite changes. Nevertheless, these changes and discomforts vary from one woman to the other.

No symptom is the same in every case, and knowing each one will help you understand what you are or will be going through once pregnant. For example, one woman may experience morning sickness while the other may not.

As for the duration of the various discomforts, they may vary as well – some may be fleeting and some may be more permanent. Most women who have undergone pregnancies have accounted for different cases. Most women start to experience discomfort during the first trimester while some experience it during the latter part of their pregnancies (third trimester).

Here are some of the more common pregnancy symptoms and discomforts pregnant women experience:

Nausea and Vomiting

Otherwise known as "morning sickness", this is one of the most common discomforts experienced during pregnancy. About 50 percent of pregnant women experience this. Ironically, this morning sickness can occur any time of the day. You could already be well-rested on your bed late at night and suddenly get this uncontrollable urge to get rid of everything you had for dinner. Alternatively, you may wake up feeling all warm and fuzzy one minute, and then feel wretched the next.

Morning sickness is due to the change in a woman's hormone levels and can be aggravated by stress or food intake. One can lessen the discomfort by eating small portions of food several times during the day. The best diet for women who experience nausea and vomiting is a diet high in complex carbohydrates. This diet includes whole-wheat food, bananas, green and leafy vegetables.

If vomiting is severe in your case, you tend to lose fluids and weight. This can lead to a condition known as hyperemesis gravidarum, which in turn can lead to dehydration. When this happens, it is important to consult your doctor. This condition may require hospitalization and rehydration via dextrose.

Fatigue

Your body changes for it to accommodate your growing baby. Because of this, your body works overtime to provide an environment conducive for the growth of the fetus. Most of the time, anemia is the underlying cause for fatigue. As the body adjusts to the pregnancy, blood volume and other fluids increase as well. With that, you can understand why pregnant women experience fatigue.

Hemorrhoids

You could develop hemorrhoids when pregnant because of the increased pressure placed on the rectum and perineum. Moreover, pregnant women are susceptible to constipation. If you experience this, consult with your doctor so she can give you the right treatment for your hemorrhoids and make recommendations on how to prevent them. For example, your doctor may suggest that you avoid sitting on the toilet for extended periods.

Breast Pain

Some women may experience breast tenderness or swelling of the breast during pregnancy. Why is this? As mentioned earlier, a woman's body goes through major changes during pregnancy to accommodate another life. The changes a woman goes through are meant to prepare her body for the pregnancy, making it a more suitable place for a baby to live in. Breasts enlarge to enable more room for milk production.

Heartburn and Indigestion

Heartburn and indigestion are caused by pressure that is placed on the intestines and stomach. This, in turn, pushes stomach content back up to the esophagus. This can be prevented by eating small meals throughout the day. In addition, avoid lying down after meals.

Yeasts Infections

During pregnancy, changes in a woman's hormone levels cause an increase in vaginal discharge. Yeast infections are most commonly characterized by thick, sticky, white discharges along with itching and irritation. Never self-medicate. Talk to your doctor and ask her how you can remedy the infection.

Pregnancy discomforts are common in every woman. The important thing is to be aware of it so that you can be prepared. Other pregnancy discomforts include:

- Stretch marks
- Constipation
- Backache
- Pica
- Fluid retention

You don't have to live through all nine months of your pregnancy in discomfort. Knowing about them and consulting with your doctor can help you manage the discomforts, making your pregnancy smoother, tolerable, and stress-free.

Chapter 5: Recommended Diet for Pregnant Women

You'll have different nutritional needs as a pregnant woman. Not only do you need additional nutrients for you changing body; you also need those nutrients for the developing baby. Having well-balanced meals during the next nine months can largely contribute toward having a healthy baby.

Having fruits and vegetables on your table should now be a daily habit. Eating at least five portions per day can go a long way. Starchy food such as rice, bread, potatoes and pasta can be beneficial especially if you tend to do a lot of physical activity, so take them regularly – but in moderate amounts.

Lean meat, chicken, fish, eggs, beans, and other protein-rich foods should make it to your pregnancy diet but only in moderation too. Even if you're craving for them, be cautious not to have too much because doing so can do more harm than good.

Calcium is equally important and you will need at least twice the regular intake. This can be obtained from foods such as milk, yoghurt, cheese and other dairy products.

Ask your physician for recommendations in vitamin supplements. Most often than not, you will be given 400 micrograms of folic acid during your first 12 weeks of pregnancy. On top of that, 10mcg of vitamin D will be necessary through the entire 9 months.

During the latter stages of pregnancy, you will probably be advised to take iron supplements as well. This is because your doctor will frequently monitor your iron levels and the supplements can be a huge help just in case you lack it. At times, special pregnancy multivitamins that contain iron, calcium, potassium, zinc, and vitamins C, D, B and E can be ideal.

Of course, you shouldn't include some foods in your pregnancy diet menu. Brie, camembert, and stilton are some cheeses you should stay away from during these periods. Besides, they contain listeria – a type of bacteria that can be harmful for your baby. Raw and uncooked meat and eggs are also a big no-no. Make sure that you cook them well before eating them. Liver and liver products typically contain too much retinol, a form of vitamin A. They can be risky for your baby in large amounts, so don't bother buying them either.

Finally, those who smoke and drink are strongly counseled to quit. It doesn't take an expert to figure out that these substances can bring undesirable consequences. Both you and your unborn baby can potentially experience health problems if you persist. Among the negative effects of smoking on babies are low birth weight, premature birth, breathing difficulties, ear infections, bronchitis, or even SIDS (sudden infant death syndrome). On the other hand, drinking can cause abnormal behavioral development, facial formalities, and other birth defects.

For more information about proper pregnancy diet, consult with your doctor regularly. Monthly visits are essential so they can know about your medical history and current condition. That way, they can prescribe specific medications that are proper for pregnant women. In addition, they may also advise you about what food to avoid in the following months.

Here's the thing, though. Pregnancy is never easy, and these words are not meant to scare you. It's a fact. There is such a thing as high-risk pregnancy, and if you want to experience the joys of motherhood, you need to know when a pregnancy is considered high-risk. The next chapter, lengthy as it is, provides you with a concise take on the subject.

Chapter 6: What Is a High Risk Pregnancy?

There have been astounding developments in medical technology. Still, I cannot emphasize enough that pregnancy could be risky. There are even some pregnancies that are way riskier than usual.

If you are a first-time mom, you are probably wondering about what some high-risk pregnancy factors are. Here are some of the common examples:

- Repeated miscarriages
- Gestational diabetes
- Type I diabetes
- Pregnancy-induced hypertension
- Problems in the placenta
- Preeclampsia and eclampsia
- Chronic hypertension
- Past or current history of preterm labor
- Multiple births (giving birth to twins, triplets, or higher)
- Various other factors as determined by your doctors

These and many more may put a woman at higher risk during her pregnancy. If you were already pregnant or still planning for it soon, this would mean seeing more than just your regular obstetrician. This means seeking the help and advice of a perinatologist, a doctor that specializes in high-risk pregnancy.

The entire experience could be overwhelming, as you would have to go to more prenatal visits. There would also be more tests as well as close monitoring of the fetus. Most of the time, both your obstetrician and perinatologist will require you to go on full bed rest, hospitalization, and other treatment options.

Pregnancies that are high risk do not necessarily mean that women with the condition would have a difficult time during labor and delivery. Most often than not, the risk is restricted during the entire course of the pregnancy. Therefore, your doctors would need to work doubly hard to ensure that they resolve any serious problems before you give birth. Nevertheless, there is what people call high-risk pregnancy complications. These conditions may occur during or after the pregnancy.

One such complication is Intrauterine Growth Restriction or IUGR. This is a condition where the fetus is smaller than normal for a few weeks during the pregnancy. You would think that a baby hasn't quite reached the full gestation age because of this condition even if it has reached full term already. A sign of this is if the baby weighs less than 90% of other fetuses at full term.

Another complication is the Rh Disease, which occurs when the blood type of the mother and that of the baby are incompatible. Everyone has a blood type and an Rh factor which can be positive or negative. If a mother is an Rh negative and the baby is Rh positive, for example, complications may arise if the baby's red blood cells end up crossing to the Rh-negative mother. This normally happens during delivery when the placenta detaches or when a pregnant woman suffers a miscarriage or goes through an abortion. Women who are most likely to experience all these are those who are within the high-risk pregnancy age bracket, 35-40 years old.

Again, reducing the risks of pregnancy requires your cooperation. Following the counsels of your doctors is crucial. They will recommend specific treatments and medication for you to experience lesser danger during your three trimesters. Make it a commitment to eat healthy meals and to avoid any food that your physician prohibits.

What Is Preeclampsia in Pregnancy?

So what is preeclampsia? This condition, which is also known as toxemia, is life threatening and normally occurs late in the second or third trimester of pregnancy. In isolated cases, preeclampsia affects postnatal women during the first six weeks after giving birth. What's difficult about this condition is it attacks unexpectedly. The only plausible symptoms are protein in a pregnant woman's urine and high blood pressure. However, sudden weight gain (one that occurs over a short period), fluid retention, headaches, and vision problems could be some of the common signs, too.

Statistics show that approximately eight percent of pregnant women suffer from preeclampsia. This and two other conditions, eclampsia and PIH or Pregnancy-Induced Hypertension, are the usual culprits behind maternal and infantile deaths. Preeclampsia in pregnancy is at its most risky if a pregnant woman doesn't even feel any of the above-mentioned signs or symptoms. Therefore, if you are expecting, it would do you good to visit your obstetrician for prenatal checkups regularly. Through regular visits, your doctor would be able to diagnose the condition. It's normally every obstetrician's standard to check or screen for symptoms of preeclampsia by keeping tabs on your weight, taking your blood pressure, or checking your urine for protein.

Edema or swelling, which is a normal occurrence during pregnancy, may actually be a sign of preeclampsia, too. Never take it for granted in case you notice any swelling on your hands and face. Go to your doctor and have her check your blood pressure. You may not be aware about it but hypertension may actually be causing the swelling. If your blood pressure reads over 140/90, then that is a cause for concern.

So who are predisposed to suffering from preeclampsia in pregnancy? Well, women who are pregnant for the first time have a higher risk of developing this condition. In addition, if a pregnant woman has a history of hypertension, diabetes, and lupus, then these put her at risk. Having other family members who suffered from preeclampsia in the past as well as multiple births may also increase the risk of this condition. At the same time, scientists are looking into the possibility that an abnormally situated placenta may be one of the reasons why pregnant women develop preeclampsia.

Once a pregnant woman is diagnosed with preeclampsia, her obstetrician will do everything possible to closely monitor her and her baby. When the baby has reached the point where it can be delivered safely, the mother would be subjected to either induced labor or birth through Caesarean section. Obviously, birth is the only cure for preeclampsia. Hence, if you were in the early stages of your pregnancy, it would be a good idea to consult your obstetrician and have her monitor your condition to detect the condition right away.

Make it a point to visit your doctor on a regular basis. Never skip on your monthly appointments because it is highly important that your doctor be always updated about your condition. Develop the habit of eating healthy foods and reserve time for exercise, as appropriate. Your doctor may tell you too many do's and don'ts but keep in mind that observing them will be for your best benefit.

Chapter 7: Pregnancy Keepsakes

For moms, nothing bets the joy of seeing their baby for the first time after taking carrying new life in their tummy for a whole 9 months! This joy is the reason that some expectant mothers create keepsakes of their pregnancies such as videos and journals.

Why Should You Start a Pregnancy Journal?

Pregnancy is certainly one of those milestones in life that can account for a woman's physical, mental, and emotional change. The notion is surreal. Inside your body, another life is growing, every inch a part of that woman's body but very much separate once it comes out after three trimesters. For most women, pregnancy is both scary and awe-inspiring.

If you were a mere observer, the pregnancy cycle would already blow your mind. Nevertheless, if you were the one carrying the child inside you, the desire to document this wonderful revelation would surely drive you to make keepsakes. That's why it's a good idea to start a pregnancy journal as soon as your obstetrician confirms the pregnancy.

Of course, there are women who start their journals post-pregnancy. However, there are more than enough reasons that one should start writing journal entries during the early stages of pregnancy. For one thing, it is during this span of time when you and your baby are growing together, literally, as one. What better way to keep all those moments in tact than with a journal, right?

Well, whatever you note down could be valuable reference in case you plan to get pregnant again in the future. On top of that, the information can be useful whenever you visit your doctor. You will be able to describe how you feel in detail.

With a journal, you can relive the pregnancy and other things with your child after you have given birth. Children are naturally curious. At some point, your kid would ask you things about what it was like when you had him or her in your tummy, among other things. Your journal would serve as some sort of storybook that you and your kid could look back on together. At this point, you probably want to know how best to start with your journal. You can always go for your gut feel, but here are a few pregnancy journal ideas you can use.

You can buy one that's readymade. You can find a plethora of pregnancy journals in bookstores. These journals usually have different features that cater to a pregnant woman's specific needs. All you have to do is look for one that fits your budget. If you have a creative flair, you can make the journal yourself. This is even better, given that you can customize the journal in such a way that allows you to write down your thoughts comfortably. You can design it any way you want; making sure that the design of the journal conveys your innermost thoughts, feelings, and personal style.

They say that pictures paint a thousand words, and if this is true, then you can document your pregnancy with pictures. You can create a pregnancy journal scrapbook, making use of scrapbooking elements and other miscellaneous items that would make your journal alive. You could even start an online journal in the form of a blog. The possibilities are endless. What's important is that you would be able to record every minute detail of your pregnancy and be able to preserve the memories of your pregnancy for posterity's sake.

What Can You Accomplish with a Pregnancy Video?

Some women, especially first-time mothers, become very overwhelmed by the news that they are pregnant to the point that they have no idea what they're supposed to do. Nevertheless, as soon as the overwhelming feeling subsides, it is immediately replaced by great excitement and increased anticipation. Most women even document their pregnancies by recording pregnancy videos. In a way, a video works the same way as a pregnancy journal does – it aims to record the entire duration of the pregnancy in living color. Of course, there are those who use the video to announce a pregnancy. With today's technology, putting the video on the internet and making it viral is no longer difficult.

Even if you've never made a video of yourself before, you would find the idea of creating a video of your pregnancy very fun. Moreover, it's a unique way to save, share, and relive various aspects of your pregnancy. With a video, you would be able to bond with your child after childbirth. You can show your child what went on after he or she was conceived, leading up to the time of his or her birth.

The idea is surreal. Some people also believe that women pregnancy video can be a wonderful expression of love. Indeed, storing everything about your pregnancy in a video that you and your family can go back to every so often is a good thing. Furthermore, a video of your 9-month journey is likely to be passed down as a memento from one generation to another.

You don't even have to be an expert in order to pull this one off. In fact, a video is one of the easiest and most fun ways to document your pregnancy. All you need is a good camera and you will be good to go. You could shoot video journals week by week. A good time to start is the first time that your obstetrician officially confirms your pregnancy.

Journals, scrapbooks, and albums still rank among the top methods used by women when it comes to pregnancy keepsakes. However, with the advent of technology, a video makes for an easy and convenient option. The process of taking pregnancy videos is extremely easy, especially since there are numerous free programs that you can use to create and to enhance the video.

Conclusion

Thank you again for downloading this book!

I hope this book was able to help you understand pregnancy better – the excitement, joy, anxiety, wonder, and uncertainty it brings to every first-time parents. Hopefully, this book helped you prepare for a new milestone in your life.

The next step is to follow the simple guidelines provided in this book to make your pregnancy safe, comfortable, and worry-free.

Finally, if you enjoyed this book, then I'd like to ask you for a favor, would you be kind enough to leave a review for this book on Amazon? It'd be greatly appreciated!

Thank you and good luck!